Let's Go with Keto

Fantastic Keto Dinner Recipes That Are Simple And Guilt Free

Copyright © 2021

All rights reserved.

DEDICATION

Contents

Keto Mac & Cheese

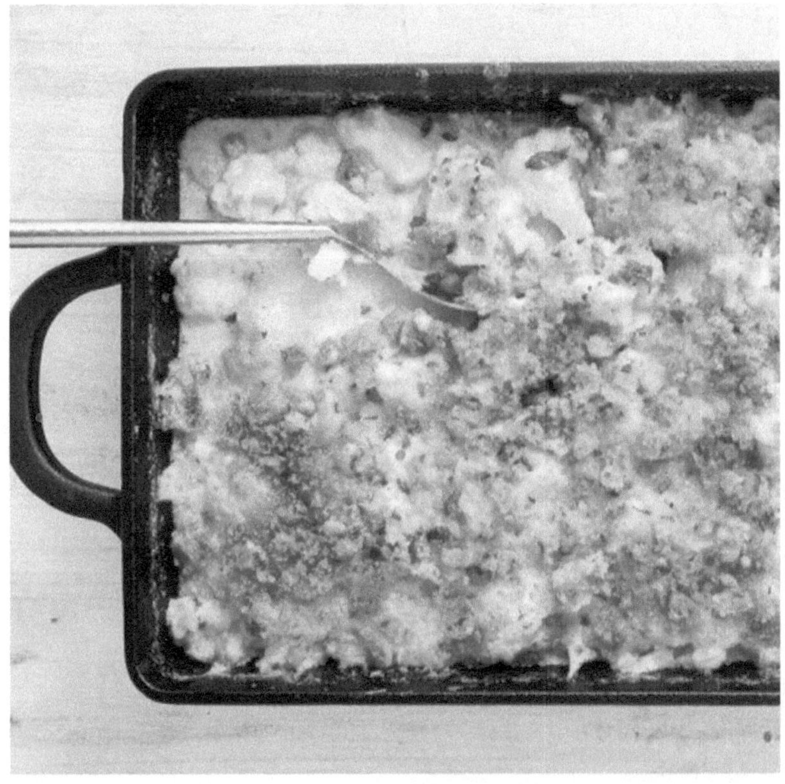

If you're keto, you know there are a lot of no-nos in classic mac & cheese. This version takes out all the trouble children (ahem, PASTA) without sacrificing flavor. The pork rind topping is totally optional, but we think it adds a pleasant crunch.

Got leftovers? Stored in an airtight container in the refrigerator, this mac will last 3 to 5 days. To reheat, we suggest popping it in a 400° oven until warmed through—the high temperature will help crisp up the topping.

INGREDIENTS

FOR THE MAC & CHEESE

Butter, for baking dish

2 medium heads cauliflower, cut into florets

2 tbsp. extra-virgin olive oil

Kosher salt

1 c. heavy cream

6 oz. cream cheese, cut into cubes

4 c. shredded cheddar

2 c. shredded mozzarella

1 tbsp. hot sauce (optional)

Freshly ground black pepper

FOR THE TOPPING

4 oz. pork rinds, crushed

1/4 c. freshly grated Parmesan

1 tbsp. extra-virgin olive oil

2 tbsp. freshly chopped parsley, for garnish

DIRECTIONS

Preheat oven to 375° and butter a 9"-x-13" baking dish. In a large bowl, toss cauliflower with 2 tablespoons oil and season with salt. Spread cauliflower onto two large baking sheets and roast until tender and lightly golden, about 40 minutes.

Meanwhile, in a large pot over medium heat, heat cream. Bring up to a simmer, then decrease heat to low and stir in cheeses until melted. Remove from heat, add hot sauce if using and season with salt and pepper, then fold in roasted cauliflower. Taste and season more if needed.

Transfer mixture to prepared baking dish. In a medium bowl stir to combine pork rinds, Parmesan, and oil. Sprinkle mixture in an even layer over cauliflower and cheese.

Bake until golden, 15 minutes. If desired, turn oven to broil to toast topping further, about 2 minutes.

Garnish with parsley before serving.

Keto Stuffed Cabbage

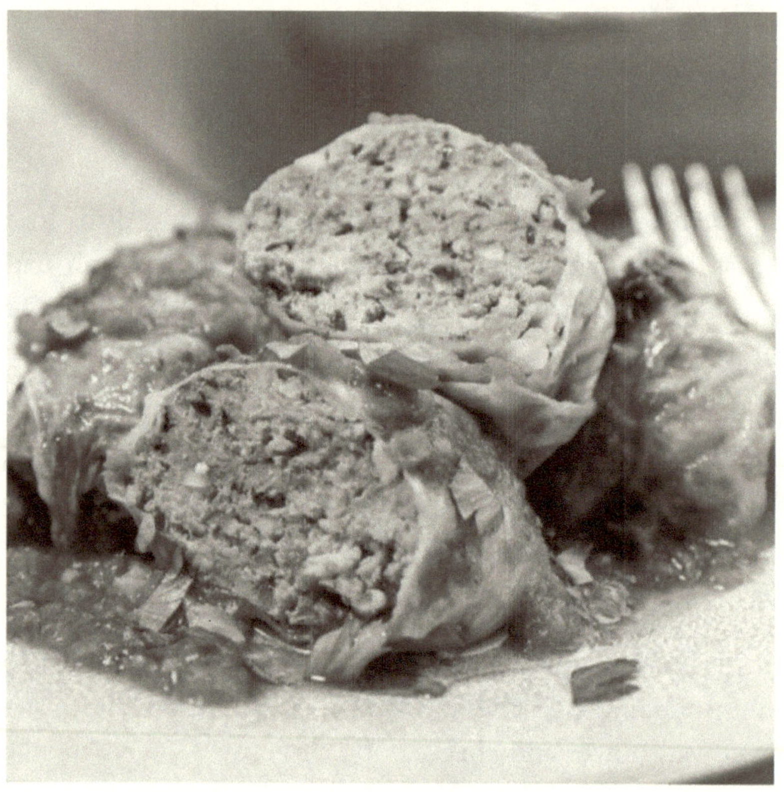

This low-carb version of stuffed cabbage is just as satisfying as the original. The secret: cauliflower rice. Homemade riced cauliflower is extremely easy, but you could also buy it pre-made.

INGREDIENTS

FOR THE SAUCE:

1 (14-oz.) can diced tomatoes

1 tbsp. apple cider vinegar

1/2 tsp. red pepper flakes

1 tsp. onion powder

1 tsp. garlic powder

1 tsp. dried oregano

Kosher salt

Freshly ground black pepper

1/4 c. extra-virgin olive oil

FOR THE CABBAGE ROLLS:

12 cabbage leaves

1 lb. ground beef

3/4 lb. ground pork

1 c. riced cauliflower

3 green onions, thinly sliced

1/4 c. chopped parsley, plus more for serving

Freshly ground black pepper

DIRECTIONS

FOR THE SAUCE:

Preheat oven to 375°. Puree tomatoes, apple cider vinegar, red pepper flakes, onion powder, garlic powder, and oregano in a blender; season with salt and pepper.

In a large deep skillet (or large pot) over medium heat, heat oil. Add pureed tomato sauce, bring to a simmer, then lower to medium-low and simmer for 20 minutes, until slightly thickened.

FOR THE CABBAGE ROLLS:

In a large pot of boiling water, blanch cabbage leaves until tender and flexible, about 1 minute. Set aside.

Make filling: in a large bowl, combine ½ c. tomato sauce, ground meats, cauliflower rice, scallions, and parsley. Season with salt and pepper.

Spread a thin layer of sauce on the bottom of a large baking dish. Using a paring knife, cut out the hard triangular rib from each cabbage leaf. Place about ⅓ cup filling into one end of each leaf, then roll up, tucking in the sides as you roll. Place rolls seam side-down on top of sauce in baking dish. Spoon remaining sauce on top of cabbage rolls. Bake 45 minutes to 55 minutes, until the meat is cooked through and internal temperature reaches 150°"

Garnish with more parsley before serving.

Keto Beef Stew

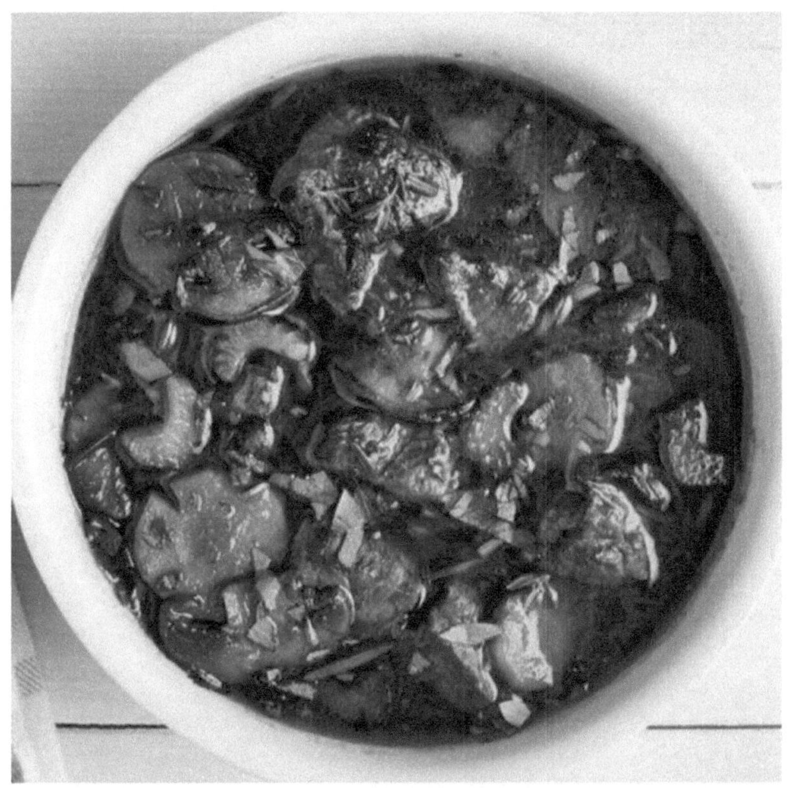

Making beef stew Keto friendly only meant a couple simple swaps. It's still silky and deeply comforting. It can make any winter night bearable and cozy. Finish the meal with any of our easy Keto desserts.

INGREDIENTS

2 lb. beef chuck roast, cut into 1" pieces

Kosher salt

Freshly ground black pepper

2 tbsp. extra-virgin olive oil

8 oz. Baby bella mushrooms, sliced

1 small onion, chopped

1 medium carrot, peeled and cut into rounds

2 stalks celery, sliced

3 cloves garlic, minced

1 tbsp. tomato paste

6 c. low-sodium beef broth

1 tsp. fresh thyme leaves

1 tsp. freshly chopped rosemary

DIRECTIONS

Pat beef dry with paper towels and season well with salt and pepper. In a large pot over medium heat, heat oil. Working in batches, add beef and sear on all sides until golden, about 3 minutes per side. Remove from pot and repeat with remaining beef, adding more oil as necessary.

To same pot, add mushrooms and cook until golden and crispy, 5 minutes. Add onion, carrots, and celery and cook until soft, 5 minutes. Add garlic and cook until fragrant, 1 minute more. Add tomato paste and and stir to coat vegetables.

Add broth, thyme, rosemary, and beef to pot and season with salt and pepper. Bring to a boil and reduce heat to a simmer. Simmer until beef is tender, 50 minutes to an hour.

Keto Corned Beef & Cabbage

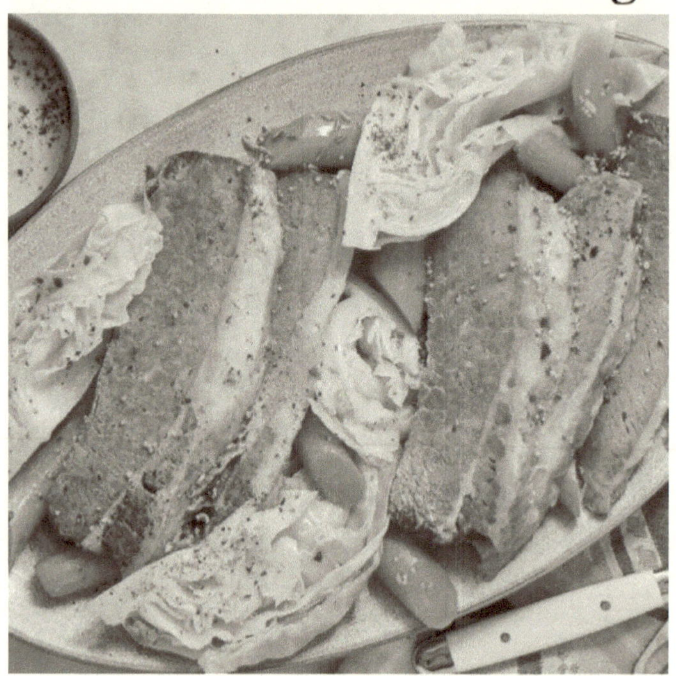

Corned beef and cabbage is a St. Patricks day MUST. This keto version is so tender and flavorful, we want to have it way more than just once a year. (Okay, the caper mayo doesn't hurt either.)

INGREDIENTS

3-4 lbs corned beef

2 onions, quartered

4 celery stalks, quartered crosswise

1 package pickling spices

Kosher salt

Black pepper

1 medium green cabbage, cut into 2" wedges

2 carrots, peeled and cut into 2" pieces

1/2 c. Dijon mustard

2 tbsp. apple cider vinegar

1/4 c. mayonnaise

2 tbsp. capers, roughly chopped, plus 1 tsp brine

2 tbsp. parsley, roughly chopped

DIRECTIONS

Place corned beef, onion, celery, and pickling spices into a large pot. Add enough water to cover by 2", season with salt and pepper, and bring to a boil. Reduce heat to low, cover, and simmer until very tender, 3–3 1/2 hours.

Meanwhile, whisk dijon mustard and apple cider vinegar in a small bowl and season with salt and pepper. In another bowl, mix mayo, capers, caper brine, and parsley. Season with salt and pepper

Add cabbage and carrots and continue to simmer for 45 minutes to 1 hour more, until cabbage is tender. Remove meat, cabbage, and carrots from pot. Slice corned beef and season with more salt and pepper.

Serve with both sauces on the side for dipping.

Keto Meatloaf

Not only is this a keto-friendly dinner, it's a much needed revamp. Everyone, including those who are not afraid of carbs, will love this bacon-wrapped meatloaf recipe. The bacon makes it insanely flavorful, the almond flour acts as the perfect binder, and the soy sauce? It packs a punch of umami you never knew you needed. Trust us, you won't miss the bread crumbs or ketchup.

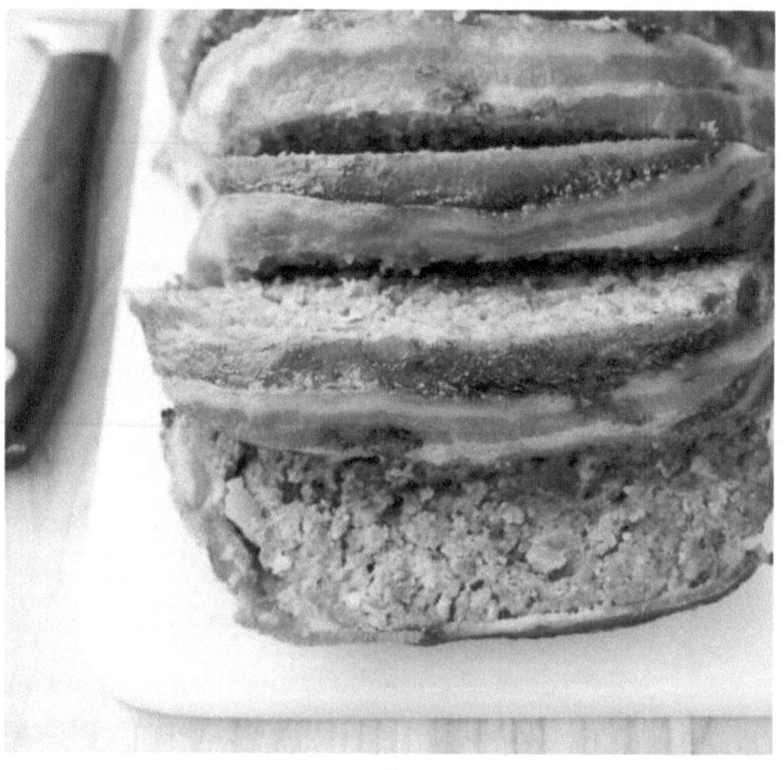

INGREDIENTS

Cooking spray

1 tbsp. extra-virgin olive oil

1 medium onion, chopped

1 stalk celery, chopped

3 cloves garlic, minced

1 tsp. dried oregano

1 tsp. chili powder

2 lb. ground beef

1 c. shredded cheddar

1/2 c. almond flour

1/4 c. grated Parmesan

2 eggs

1 tbsp. low-sodium soy sauce

Kosher salt

Freshly ground black pepper

6 thin strips bacon

DIRECTIONS

Preheat oven to 400°. Grease a medium baking dish with cooking spray. In a medium skillet over medium heat, heat oil. Add onion and celery and cook until soft, 5 minutes. Stir in garlic, oregano, and chili powder and cook until fragrant, 1 minute. Let mixture cool slightly.

In a large bowl, combine ground beef, vegetable mixture, cheese, almond flour, Parmesan, eggs, soy sauce, and season with salt and pepper. Shape into a large loaf in baking dish, then lay bacon slices on top.

Cook until bacon is crispy and beef is cooked through, about 1 hour. If bacon is cooking too quickly, cover dish with foil.

Keto Chicken Parmesan

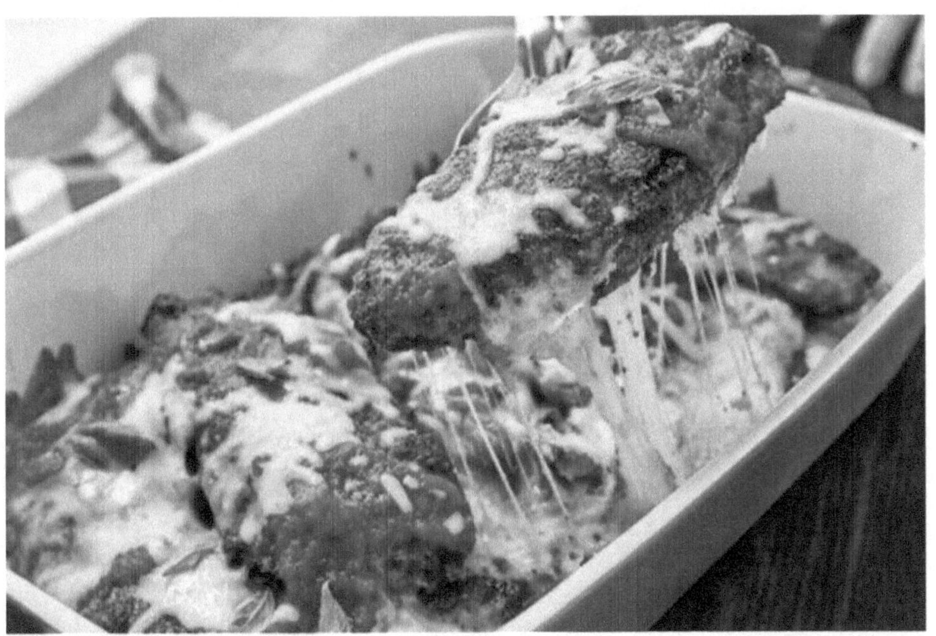

INGREDIENTS

4 boneless skinless chicken breasts

Kosher salt

Freshly ground black pepper

1 c. almond flour

3 large eggs, beaten

3 c. freshly grated Parmesan, plus more for serving

2 tsp. garlic powder

1 tsp. onion powder

2 tsp. dried oregano

Vegetable oil

3/4 c. low-carb sugar-free tomato sauce

1 1/2 c. shredded mozzarella

Fresh basil leaves, for topping

DIRECTIONS

Preheat oven to 400°. Using a sharp knife, cut chicken breasts in half crosswise. Season chicken on both sides with salt and pepper.

Place eggs and almond flour in 2 separate shallow bowls. In a third shallow bowl, combine Parmesan, garlic powder, onion powder, and oregano. Season with salt and pepper.

Working with one at a time, dip chicken cutlets into almond flour, then eggs, and then Parmesan mixture, pressing to coat.

In a large skillet over medium heat, heat 2 tablespoons oil. Add chicken and cook until golden and cooked through, 2 to 3 minutes per side. Work in batches as necessary, adding more oil when needed.

Transfer fried cutlets to a 9"-x-13" baking dish, evenly spread tomato sauce on each cutlet and top with mozzarella.

Bake until cheese is melty, 10 to 12 minutes. If desired, broil until cheese is golden, 3 minutes.

Top with basil and more Parmesan before serving.

Keto Taco Casserole

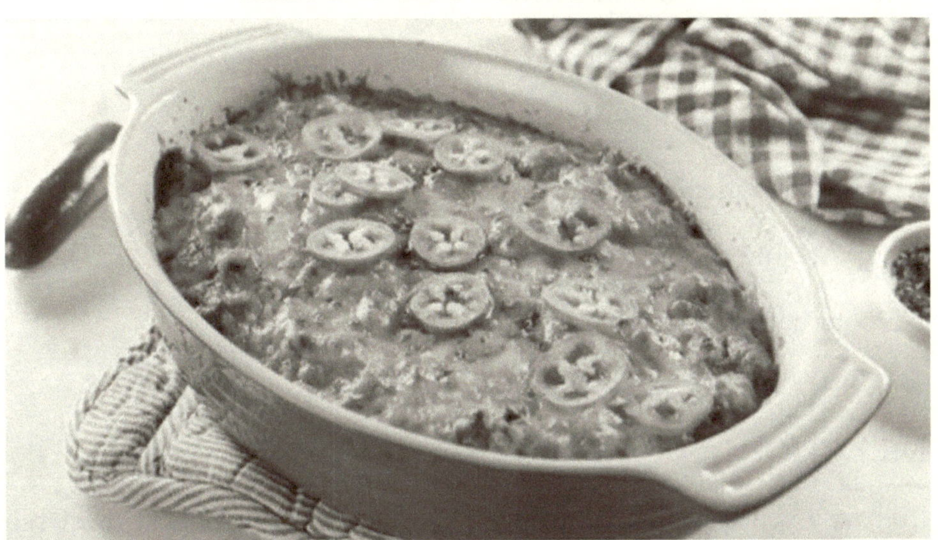

Keto people, meet your new favorite weeknight dinner. It's super-easy, extremely hearty, and it's got a little kick from the jalapeño. We packed all of your favorite Tex-Mex flavors into this endlessly scoopable and delicious casserole. Make a batch of keto tortilla chips and you won't need any utensils, simply dip and chow down. Finish off with our keto frosty for a decadent and delicious keto feast!

INGREDIENTS

1 tbsp. extra-virgin olive oil

1/2 yellow onion, diced

2 lb. ground beef

2 tbsp. kosher salt

Freshly ground black pepper

2 tbsp. keto taco seasoning mix

1 jalapeño, seeded and minced, plus more sliced for garnish

6 large eggs, lightly beaten

2 c. shredded Mexican cheese

2 tbsp. freshly chopped parsley leaves

1 c. sour cream, for serving (optional)

DIRECTIONS

Preheat oven to 350°. In a large skillet over medium heat, heat oil. Add onion and cook until slightly softened, 2 minutes.

Add ground beef and season with salt and pepper. Cook, breaking up meat with a wooden spoon, until no longer pink, 6 minutes. Sprinkle in taco seasoning and jalapeño and cook, stirring, until spices are lightly toasted, 1 minute. Drain and let cool slightly.

In a large mixing bowl, whisk eggs, then add in meat mixture. Spread mixture into an even layer in the bottom of a 2-quart baking dish. Sprinkle with cheese.

Bake until set, about 25 minutes.

Sprinkle with parsley and top each slice with a dollop of sour cream and jalapeño, if desired.

Keto Bacon Sushi

Being on a keto diet means you have way fewer options for snacking. Never fear! These little guys will satisfy all your snack cravings: They're salty, creamy, and crunchy, but they won't weigh you down. We went for carrots, cucumbers, and avocado for our filling, but the options are endless. Switch it up with bell peppers, celery, radishes, or whatever else you have on hand!

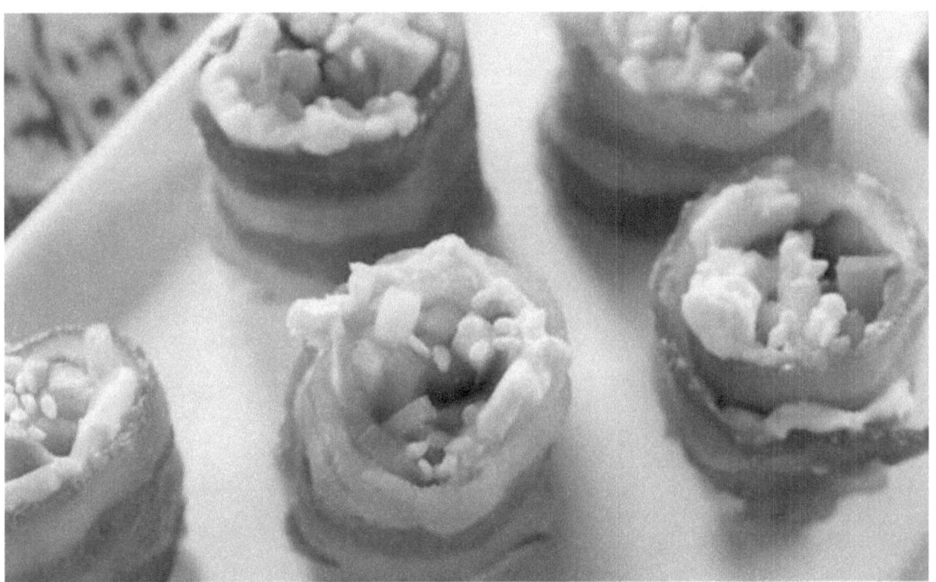

INGREDIENTS

6 slices bacon, halved

2 Persian cucumbers, thinly sliced

2 medium carrots, thinly sliced

1 avocado, sliced

4 oz. cream cheese, softened

Sesame seeds, for garnish

DIRECTIONS

Preheat oven to 400°. Line a baking sheet with aluminum foil and fit it with a cooling rack. Lay bacon halves in an even layer and bake until slightly crisp but still pliable, 11 to 13 minutes.

Meanwhile, cut cucumbers, carrots, and avocado into sections roughly the width of the bacon.

When bacon is cool enough to touch, spread an even layer of cream cheese on each slice. Divide vegetables evenly between the bacon and place on one end. Roll up vegetables tightly.

Garnish with sesame seeds and serve.

Keto Meatballs

Extra cheese holds these tender meatballs together perfectly without any type of flour. A breeze to whip up makes these the perfect weeknight dinner for everyone and leaving you plenty of time whip up a Keto Cheesecake for dessert! We use all ground beef in these meatballs, but they work well with other types of ground meat as well. Ground turkey and ground pork both are great or a combination of ground pork and beef makes for exceptional meatballs. To make these extra tender, handle them as little as possible. Just like a cake, the more you mix and mess with meatballs, the tougher they become! If you find these hard to form at all because of the lack of breadcrumbs, wet your hands slightly to help keep them from sticking to your hands.

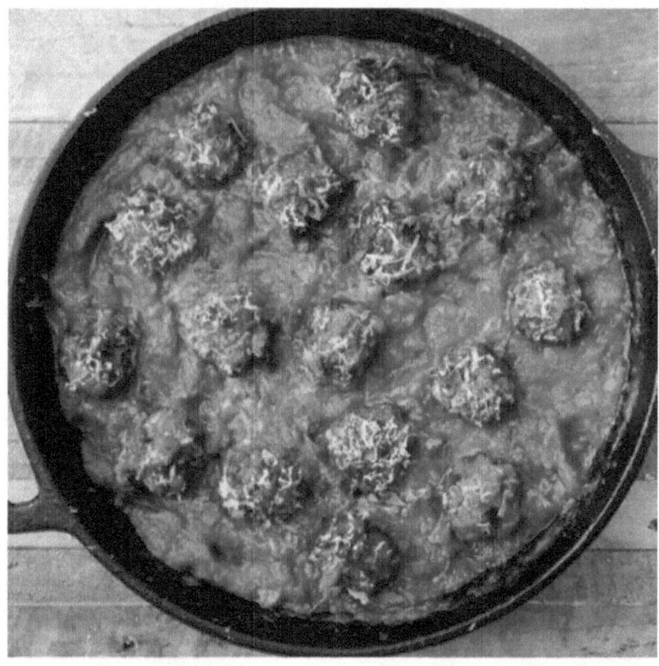

INGREDIENTS

FOR THE MEATBALLS

1 lb. ground beef

1 clove garlic, minced

1/2 c. shredded mozzarella

1/4 c. freshly grated Parmesan, plus more for serving

2 tbsp. freshly chopped parsley

1 large egg, beaten

1 tsp. kosher salt

1/2 tsp. freshly ground black pepper

2 tbsp. extra-virgin olive oil

FOR THE SAUCE

1 medium onion, chopped

2 cloves garlic, minced

1 (28-oz.) can crushed tomatoes

1 tsp. dried oregano

Kosher salt

Freshly ground black pepper

DIRECTIONS

In a large bowl combine beef, garlic, mozzarella, Parmesan, parsley, egg, salt, and pepper. Form into 16 meatballs.

In a large skillet over medium heat, heat oil. Add meatballs and cook, turning occasionally, until golden on all sides, about 10 minutes. Remove from skillet and place on a paper towel-lined plate.

To the same skillet, add onion and cook until soft, 5 minutes. Add garlic and cook until fragrant, 1 minute more. Add tomatoes and oregano and season with salt and pepper.

Add meatballs back to skillet, cover and simmer until sauce has thickened, 15 minutes. Garnish with Parmesan before serving.

Keto Broccoli Salad

This easy broccoli salad is the perfect meal prep recipe. Besides being well-rounded and healthy, we think it's even better the next day. If you're vegetarian, swap out the bacon for a diced avocado—the creaminess is a great compliment to the snappy broccoli.

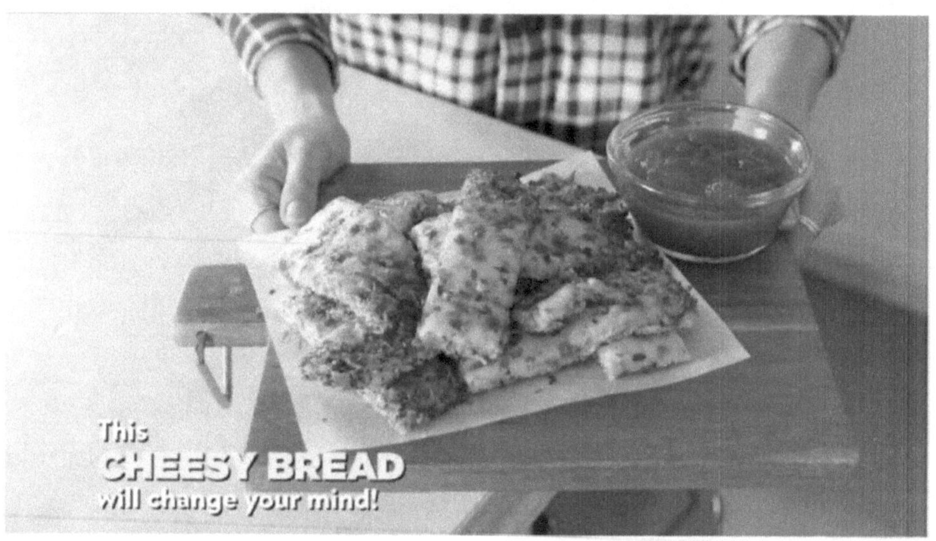

INGREDIENTS

FOR THE SALAD

kosher salt

3 heads broccoli, cut into bite-size pieces

1/2 c. shredded Cheddar

1/4 red onion, thinly sliced

1/4 c. toasted sliced almonds

3 slices bacon, cooked and crumbled

2 tbsp. freshly chopped chives

FOR THE DRESSING

2/3 c. mayonnaise

3 tbsp. apple cider vinegar

1 tbsp. dijon mustard

Kosher salt

Freshly ground black pepper

DIRECTIONS

In a medium pot or saucepan, bring 6 cups of salted water to a boil. While waiting for the water to boil, prepare a large bowl with ice water.

Add broccoli florets to the boiling water and cook until tender, 1 to 2 minutes. Remove with a slotted spoon and place in the prepared bowl of ice water. When cool, drain florets in a colander.

In a medium bowl, whisk to combine dressing ingredients. Season to taste with salt and pepper.

Combine all salad ingredients in a large bowl and pour over dressing. Toss until ingredients are combined and fully coated in dressing. Refrigerate until ready to serve.

Keto Taco Cups

Taco shells made out of cheese = the ultimate keto hack. We're basically talking about frico, an Italian cooking method in which cheese is cooked in a pan until slightly crispy but malleable. Here's we're baking little mounds of cheddar and shaping them into handheld cups.

These are not authentic or traditional tacos by any means. But, if you're a fan of Tex-Mex ground beef tacos and are trying to follow a low-carb diet, these are a fun option.

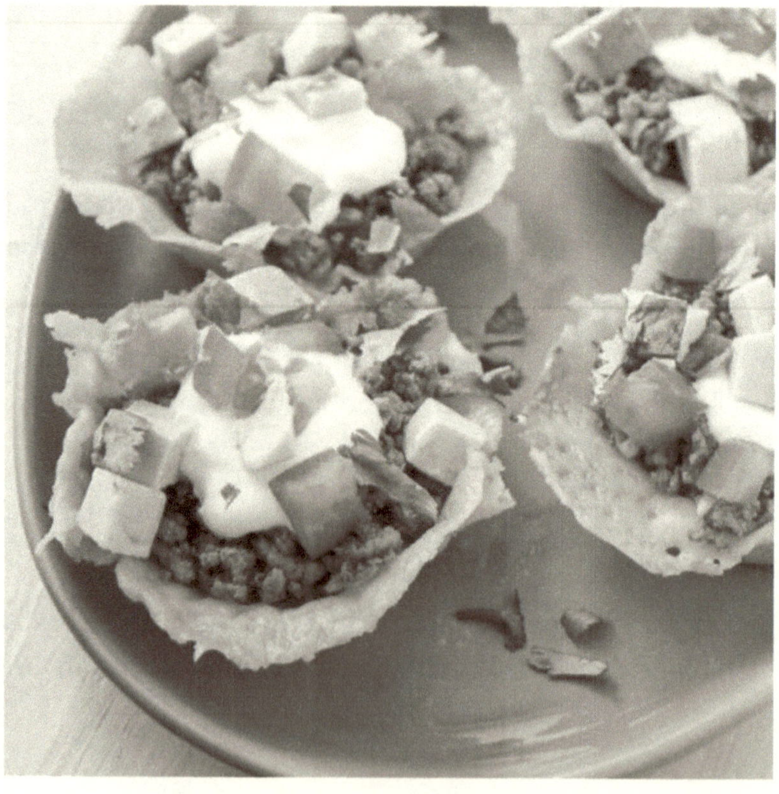

INGREDIENTS

2 c. shredded cheddar

1 tbsp. extra-virgin olive oil

1 small onion, chopped

3 cloves garlic, minced

1 lb. ground beef

1 tsp. chili powder

1/2 tsp. ground cumin

1/2 tsp. paprika

Kosher salt

Freshly ground black pepper

Sour cream, for serving

Diced avocado, for serving

Freshly chopped cilantro, for serving

Chopped tomatoes, for serving

DIRECTIONS

Preheat oven to 375° and line a large baking sheet with parchment paper. Spoon about 2 tablespoons cheddar a few inches apart. Bake until bubbly and edges are beginning to turn golden, about 6 minutes.

Let cool on baking sheet for a minute.

Meanwhile, grease bottom of a muffin tin with cooking spray, then carefully pick up melted cheese slices and place on bottom of muffin tin. Fit with another inverted muffin tin and let cool 10 minutes. If you don't have a second muffin tin, use your hands to help mold the cheese around the inverted tin.

In a large skillet over medium heat, heat oil. Add onion and cook, stirring occasionally, until softened, about 5 minutes. Stir in garlic, then add ground beef, breaking up meat with a wooden spoon. Cook until beef is no longer pink, about 6 minutes, then drain fat.

Return meat to skillet and season with chili powder, cumin, paprika, salt, and pepper.

Transfer cheese cups to a serving platter. Fill with cooked ground beef and top with sour cream, avocado, cilantro, and tomatoes.

Keto Fried Chicken

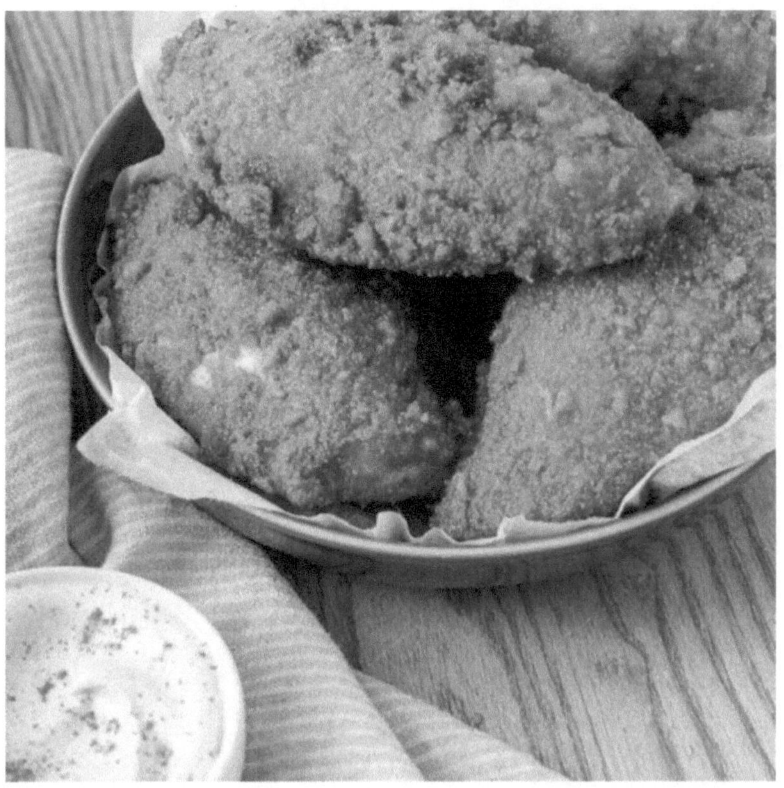

To make a Keto Friendly fried chicken we skipped the flour and went for pork rinds and Parmesan. Almond flour helps adhere everything together as well for a perfectly crisp chicken. We also baked this chicken to skip all of the unnecessary oil but it still bakes into a chicken breast that you would swear was fried. Feel free to use thighs or drumsticks as well, just know the bake time will be longer!

INGREDIENTS

FOR THE CHICKEN

6 bone-in, skin-on chicken breasts (about 4 lbs.)

Kosher salt

Freshly ground black pepper

2 large eggs

1/2 c. heavy cream

3/4 c. almond flour

1 1/2 c. finely crushed pork rinds

1/2 c. freshly grated Parmesan

1 tsp. garlic powder

1/2 tsp. paprika

FOR THE SPICY MAYO

1/2 c. mayonnaise

1 1/2 tsp. hot sauce

DIRECTIONS

Preheat oven to 400° and line a large baking sheet with parchment paper. Pat chicken dry with paper towels and season with salt and pepper.

In a shallow bowl whisk together eggs and heavy cream. In another shallow bowl, combine almond flour, pork rinds, Parmesan, garlic powder, and paprika. Season with salt and pepper.

Working one at a time, dip chicken in egg mixture and then in almond flour mixture, pressing to coat. Place chicken on prepared baking sheet.

Bake until chicken is golden and internal temperature reaches 165°, about 45 minutes.

Meanwhile make dipping sauce: In a medium bowl, combine mayonnaise and hot sauce. Add more hot sauce depending on preferred spiciness level.

Serve chicken warm with dipping sauce.

Keto Zoodle Alfredo With Bacon

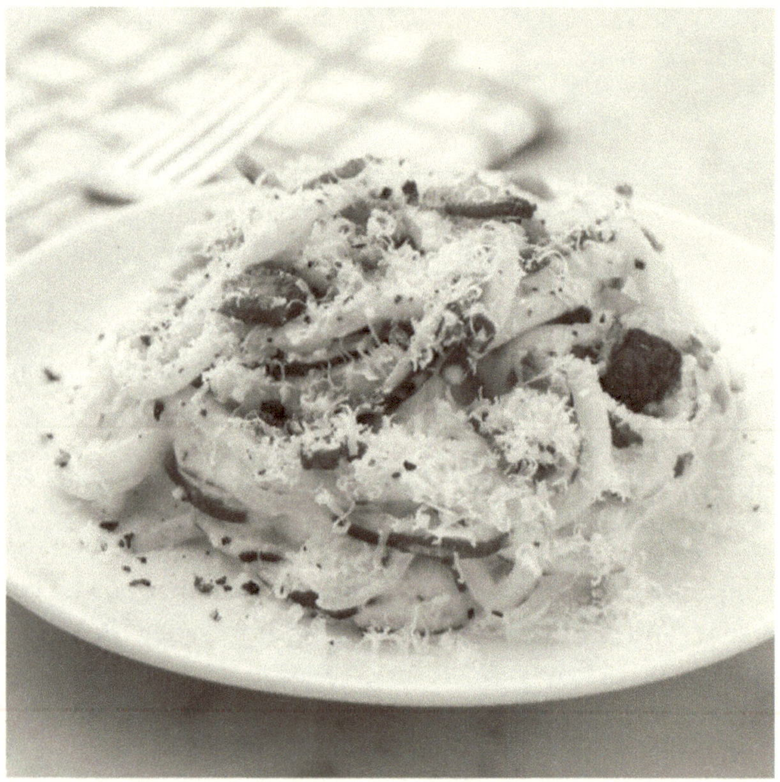

We here at Delish zoodles. Not just because we think it's such a fun word to say but also because they are a flavorful and nutritious alternative to regular pasta. This zoodle alfredo gives the original a run for it's money! That's partly because we love that its a little less of a guilty pleasure when made with zucchini but also because we load it up with tons of bacon! AND it takes just as long if not less time to make than the original. You can't afford not to make this amazing keto-friendly recipe!

INGREDIENTS

1/2 lb. bacon, chopped

1 shallot, chopped

2 cloves garlic, minced

1/4 c. white wine

1 1/2 c. heavy cream

1/2 c. grated Parmesan cheese, plus more for garnish

1 (16 oz.) container zucchini noodles

Kosher Salt

Freshly ground black pepper

DIRECTIONS

In a large skillet over medium heat, cook bacon until crispy, 8 minutes. Drain on a paper towel-lined plate.

Pour off all but 2 tablespoons of bacon, then add shallots . Cook until soft, about 2 minutes, then add the garlic and cook until fragrant, about 30 seconds. Add wine and cook until reduced by half.

Add heavy cream and bring mixture to a boil. Reduce heat to low and stir in Parmesan. Cook until sauce has thickened slightly, about 2 minutes. Add zucchini noodles and toss until completely coated in sauce. Remove from heat and stir in cooked bacon.

Keto Quesadillas

This "quesadilla" may not be a doppelgänger for the beloved Mexican dish, commonly made with corn or flour tortillas and melty cheese. BUT, when the craving strikes, this keto-fied quesadilla is so satisfying.

What makes this recipe so genius? The cheese "tortilla"! To make sure you don't have any issues removing the quesadilla from your tray, let it cool for 1 to 2 minutes. When it's slightly cool, it's much easier to separate from the parchment paper. If you've got an offset spatula, now is it's time to shine!

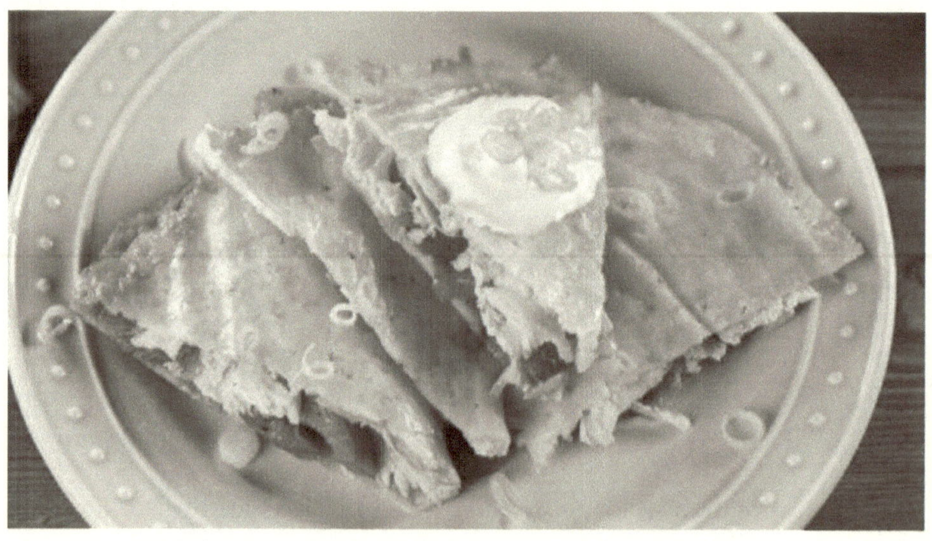

INGREDIENTS

1 tbsp. extra-virgin olive oil

1 bell pepper, sliced

35

1/2 yellow onion, sliced

1/2 tsp. chili powder

Kosher salt

Freshly ground black pepper

3 c. shredded Monterey Jack

3 c. shredded cheddar

4 c. shredded chicken

1 avocado, thinly sliced

1 green onion, thinly sliced

Sour cream, for serving

DIRECTIONS

Preheat oven to 400° and line two medium baking sheets with parchment paper.

In a medium skillet over medium-high heat, heat oil. Add pepper and onion and season with chili powder, salt, and pepper. Cook until soft, 5 minutes. Transfer to a plate.

In a medium bowl, stir together cheeses. Add 1 1/2 cups of cheese mixture into the center of both prepared baking sheets. Spread into an even layer and shape into a circle, the size of a flour tortilla.

Bake cheeses until melty and slightly golden around the edge, 8 to 10 minutes. Add onion-pepper mixture, shredded chicken, and avocado slices to one half of each. Let cool slightly, then use the parchment paper and a small spatula to gently lift and fold one side of the cheese "tortilla" over the side with the fillings. Return to oven to heat, 3 to 4 minutes more. Repeat to make 2 more quesadillas.

Cut each quesadilla into quarters. Garnish with green onion and sour cream before serving.

Keto Chili

This isn't your classic chili. There are a few ingredients (tomatoes, beans) that aren't so keto-friendly, and we chose to leave out. Don't let that stop you, though! Every diet is different, and if you feel like switching up or adding more ingredients, do you!

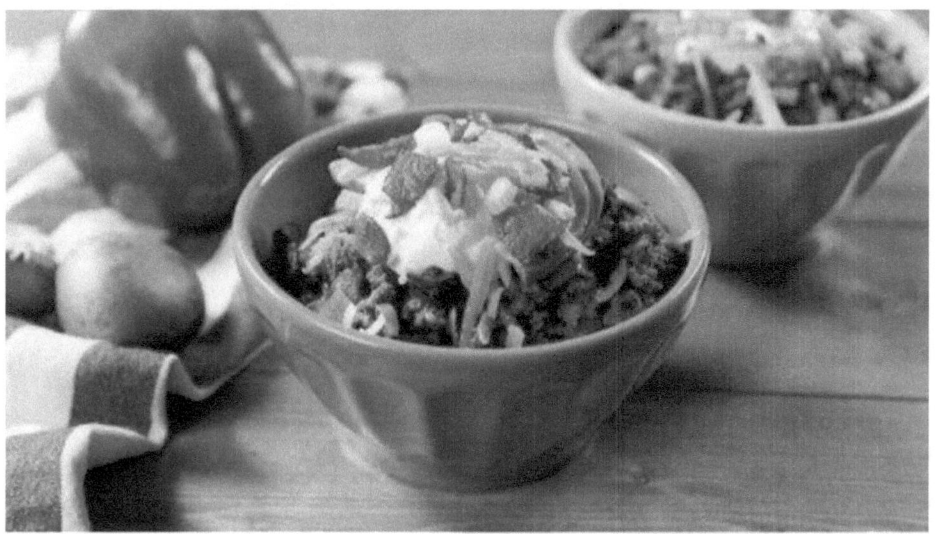

INGREDIENTS

3 slices bacon, cut into 1/2" strips

1/4 medium yellow onion, chopped

2 celery stalks, chopped

1 green bell pepper, chopped

1/2 c. sliced baby Bellas

2 cloves garlic, minced

2 lb. ground beef

2 tbsp. chili powder

2 tsp. ground cumin

2 tsp. dried oregano

2 tbsp. smoked paprika

Kosher salt

Freshly ground black pepper

2 c. low-sodium beef broth

Sour cream, for garnish

Shredded cheddar, for garnish

Sliced green onions, for garnish

Sliced avocado, for garnish

DIRECTIONS

In a large pot over medium heat, cook bacon. When bacon is crisp, remove from pot with a slotted spoon. Add onion, celery, pepper, and mushrooms to pot and cook until soft, 6 minutes. Add garlic and cook until fragrant, 1 minute more.

Push vegetables to one side of the pan and add beef. Cook, stirring occasionally, until no pink remains. Drain fat and return to heat.

Add chili powder, cumin, oregano, and paprika and season with salt and pepper. Stir to combine and cook 2 minutes more. Add broth and bring to a simmer. Let cook 10 to 15 more minutes, until most of the broth has evaporated.

Ladle into bowls and top with sour cream, reserved bacon, cheese, green onions, and avocado.

Keto Breaded Shrimp

Crushed pork rinds give shrimp a salty crunch every keto-lover will appreciate. You won't miss the bread crumbs one bit. If you're a pescatarian, don't worry — we have plenty more low-carb keto ideas up our sleeve.

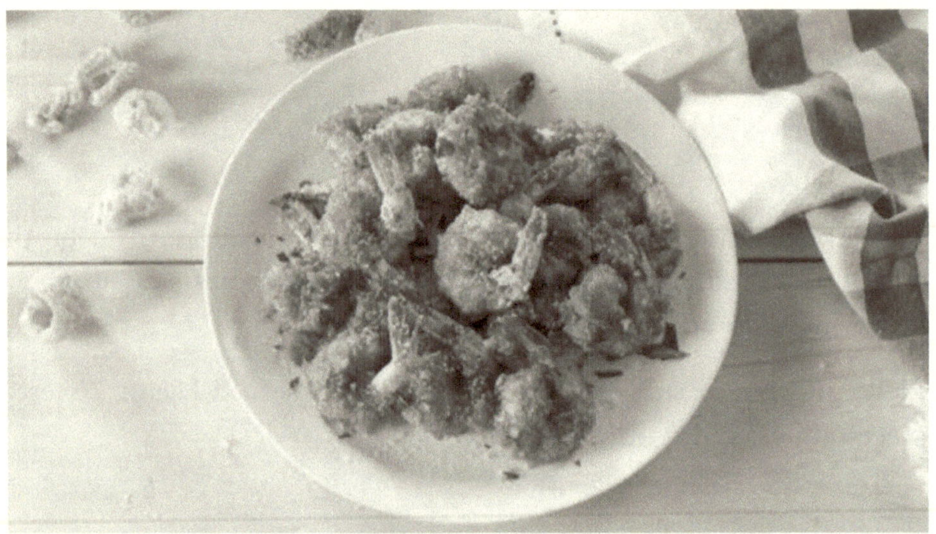

INGREDIENTS

Cooking spray

6 oz. pork rinds

1/4 c. grated Parmesan

1 tsp. chili powder

1/2 tsp. paprika

1/2 tsp. garlic powder

1/2 tsp. dried oregano

Kosher salt

2 large eggs, beaten

Freshly ground black pepper

1 lb. large shrimp

FOR THE SAUCE + GARNISH

1/2 c. mayonnaise (or sour cream)

Juice of 1/2 lemon

Dash of hot sauce

Freshly chopped parsley

DIRECTIONS

Preheat oven to 450°. Grease a large rimmed baking sheet with cooking spray. In a food processor (or in a resealable bag using a rolling pin), crush pork rinds into fine crumbs. Transfer to a medium shallow bowl and whisk in Parmesan, spices, and herbs. Season mixture with salt and pepper.

Pour beaten eggs into a small shallow bowl. Dredge shrimp in eggs, letting excess drip, then coat in pork rind mixture.

Place breaded shrimp on prepared baking sheet in single layer. Bake until coating is crispy and shrimp is cooked through, 10 to 12 minutes.

Meanwhile, make sauce: In a small bowl, whisk together mayonnaise, lemon juice, and hot sauce. Garnish shrimp with parsley and serve.

Keto Pork Chops

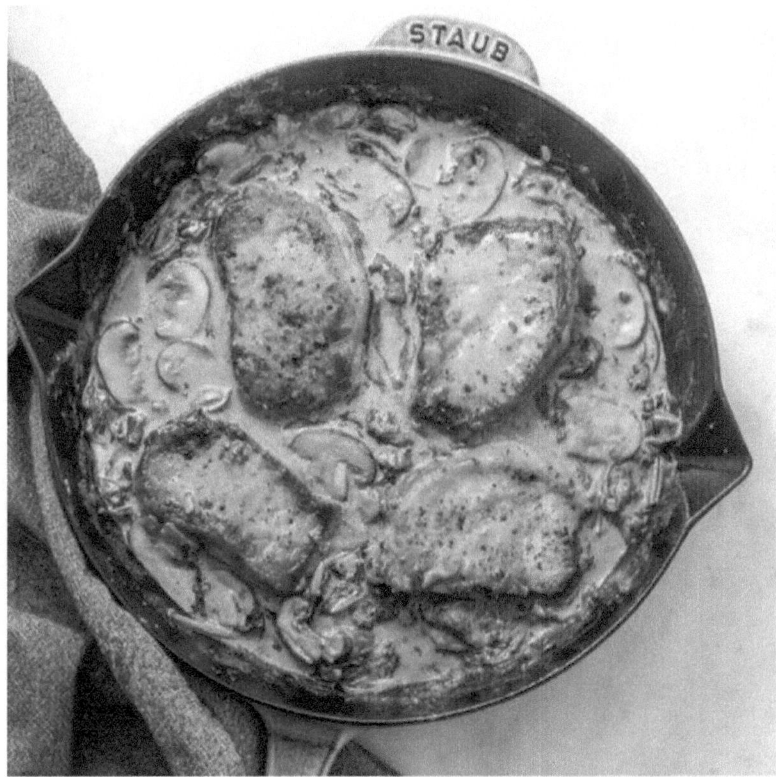

How can something this creamy and delicious be Keto!? These easy pork chops come complete with a mushroom cream sauce that you'll want to pour over everything. If all Keto dinners are this good, sign us up! The cream sauce helps keep the pork chops from tasting dried out and keeps this from being just a boring cut of pork chops. Bonus! It all comes together in well under an hour.

INGREDIENTS

4 boneless pork chops

Kosher salt

Freshly ground black pepper

2 tbsp. extra-virgin olive oil

8 oz. baby bella mushrooms, sliced

2 cloves garlic, minced

1/2 c. heavy cream

1/2 c. freshly grated Parmesan

1 tsp. dried oregano

Pinch crushed red pepper flakes

3 c. packed baby spinach

DIRECTIONS

Season pork chops on both sides with salt and pepper. In a large skillet over medium heat, heat oil. Add pork chops and cook until golden and cooked through. Remove from skillet and place on a plate to keep warm.

Add mushrooms to skillet and cook until softened, 5 minutes, then add garlic and cook until fragrant, 1 minute more.

Add heavy cream, Parmesan, oregano, and a pinch of red pepper

45

flakes. Season with salt and pepper. Bring sauce to a simmer and cook until thickened, about 3 minutes. Add spinach and cook until wilted, 2 minutes more.

Return pork chops to skillet and cook until warmed through, 5 minutes.

Keto Burger Buns

Don't skip the bun.

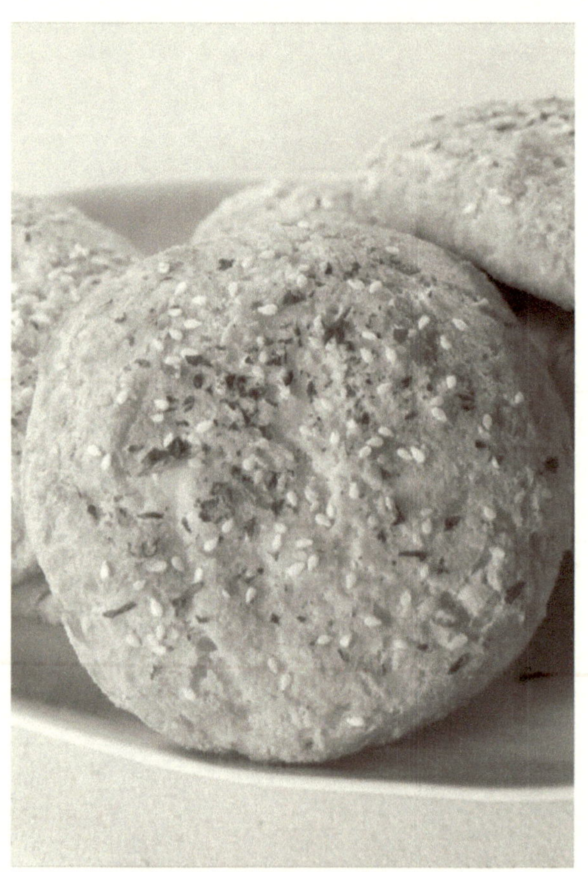

INGREDIENTS

2 c. shredded mozzarella

4 oz. cream cheese

3 large eggs

3 c. almond flour

2 tsp. baking powder

1 tsp. kosher salt

4 tbsp. butter, melted

sesame seeds Sesame

dried parsley

DIRECTIONS

Preheat oven to 400° and line a baking sheet with parchment paper. In a large microwave-safe bowl, melt together mozzarella and cream cheese.

Add eggs and stir to combine then add almond flour, baking powder and salt. Form dough into 6 balls and flatten slightly then place on prepared baking sheet.

Brush with butter and sprinkle with sesame seeds and parsley. Bake until golden, 10-12 minutes.

Keto Chicken Soup

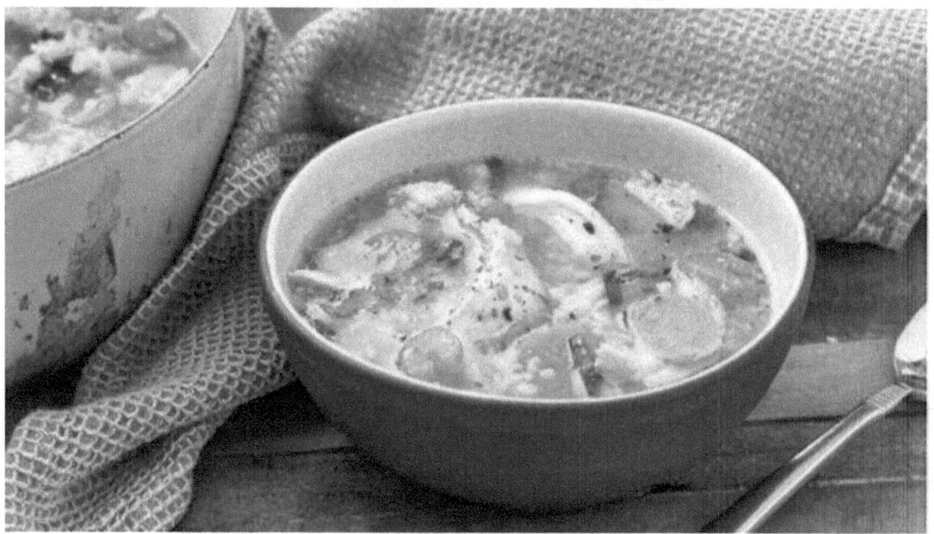

When we're sick, or hungover, or we've just eaten WAY too much junk, we always crave a simple and satisfying chicken noodle soup. Packed with veggies and protein, it's exactly what we need to get us back on track.

For those on keto, chicken noodle soup isn't exactly an option because of those pesky, carb-loaded noodles. Instead, this version gets a hearty boost with cauliflower rice, and we're big fans. Don't skimp on the ginger—it adds an irresistible kick to the broth. Serve with a squeeze of lemon or lime if you're feeling zesty.

INGREDIENTS

2 tbsp. vegetable oil

1 medium onion, chopped

5 cloves garlic, smashed

2" piece fresh ginger, sliced

1 small cauliflower, cut into florets

3/4 tsp. crushed red pepper flakes

1 medium carrot, peeled and thinly sliced on a bias

6 c. low-sodium chicken broth

1 stalk celery, thinly sliced

2 boneless skinless chicken breasts

Freshly chopped parsley, for garnish

DIRECTIONS

In a large pot over medium heat, heat oil. Add onion, garlic and ginger. Cook until beginning to brown.

Meanwhile, pulse cauliflower in a food processor until broken down into rice-sized granules. Add cauliflower to pot with onion mixture and cook over medium high heat until beginning to brown, about 8 minutes.

Add pepper flakes, carrots, celery and chicken broth and bring to a simmer. Add chicken breasts and let cook gently until they reach an internal temperature of 165°, about 15 minutes. Remove from pan, let cool until cool enough to handle, and shred. Meanwhile, continue simmering until vegetables are tender, 3 to 5 minutes more.

Remove ginger from pot, and add shredded chicken back to soup. Season to taste with salt and pepper, then garnish with parsley before serving.

Keto Burger Fat Bombs

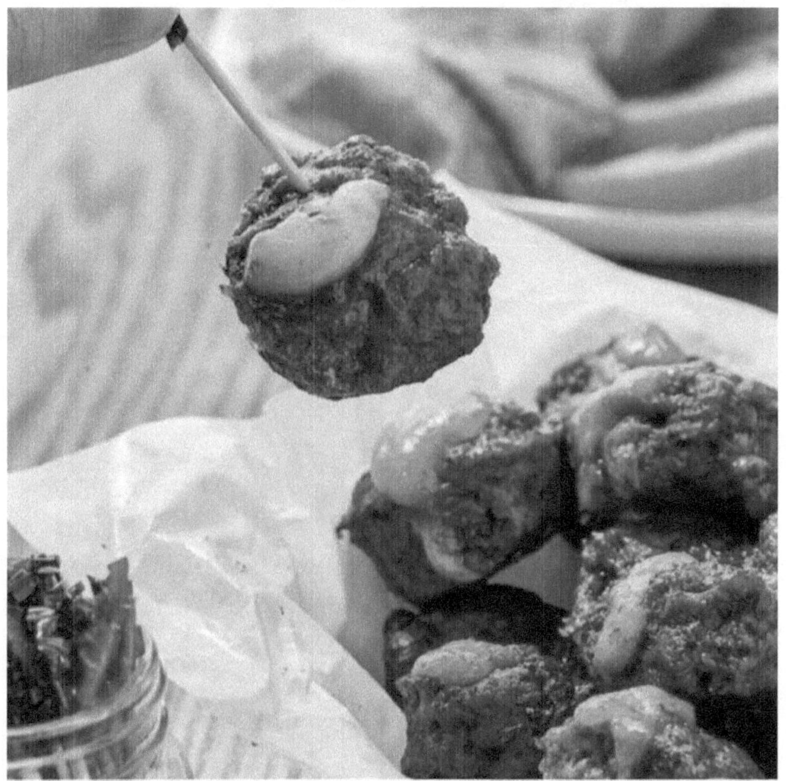

The secret ingredient in these burger fat bombs: BUTTER. It'll help keep you satisfied and happy for way longer than your favorite fast food joint ever could. Plus, cheddar is always a welcomed surprise.

INGREDIENTS

Cooking spray

1 lb. ground beef

1/2 tsp. garlic powder

Kosher salt

Freshly ground black pepper

2 tbsp. cold butter, cut into 20 pieces

2 oz. cheddar, cut into 20 pieces

Lettuce leaves, for serving

Thinly sliced tomatoes, for serving

Mustard, for serving

DIRECTIONS

Preheat oven to 375° and grease a mini muffin tin with cooking spray. In a medium bowl, season beef with garlic powder, salt, and pepper.

Press 1 teaspoon beef evenly into the bottom of each muffin tin cup, completely covering the bottom. Place a piece of butter on top then press 1 teaspoon beef over butter to completely cover.

Place a piece of cheddar on top of meat in each cup then press remaining beef over cheese to completely cover.

Bake until meat is cooked through, about 15 minutes. Let cool slightly.

Carefully, use a metal offset spatula to release each burger from the tin. Serve with lettuce leaves, tomatoes, and mustard.

Keto Dogs

We love this Keto bread recipe. It is so simple to make and is one heck of a great bread substitute.

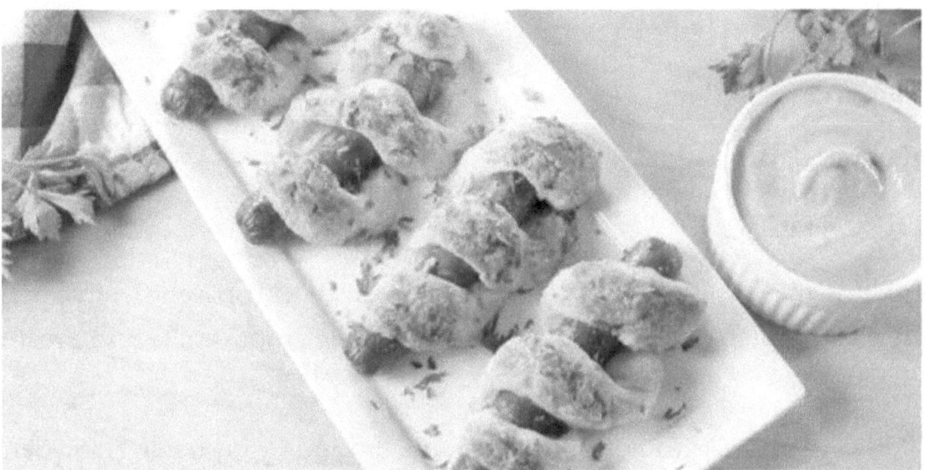

INGREDIENTS

2 c. shredded mozzarella

4 oz. cream cheese

2 large eggs, beaten

2 1/2 c. almond flour

2 tsp. baking powder

1 tsp. kosher salt

8 hot dogs

4 tbsp. butter, melted

1 tsp. garlic powder

1 tbsp. freshly chopped parsley

Mustard, for serving

DIRECTIONS

Preheat oven to 400° and line a baking sheet with parchment paper. In a large microwave-safe bowl, melt together mozzarella and cream cheese.

Add eggs and stir to combine then add almond flour, baking powder, and salt.

Divide dough into 8 balls then shape each ball into long ropes.

Wrap a rope around each hot dog.

In a small bowl whisk together butter, garlic powder, and parsley.

Brush garlic butter over each hot dog then bake until golden, 1o-15 minutes.

Serve with mustard.

Keto Pizza Chaffles

Being on the Keto diet doesn't mean you have to miss out on all of your favorite foods, especially waffles! Chaffles, or cheese waffles, make a great breakfast, lunch, or dinner. We opted to top ours with all of favorite pizza toppings but you can even leave these plain and top them with the classic butter and syrup (Keto-friendly, of course). The cheese ensures these crisp up to absolute perfection.

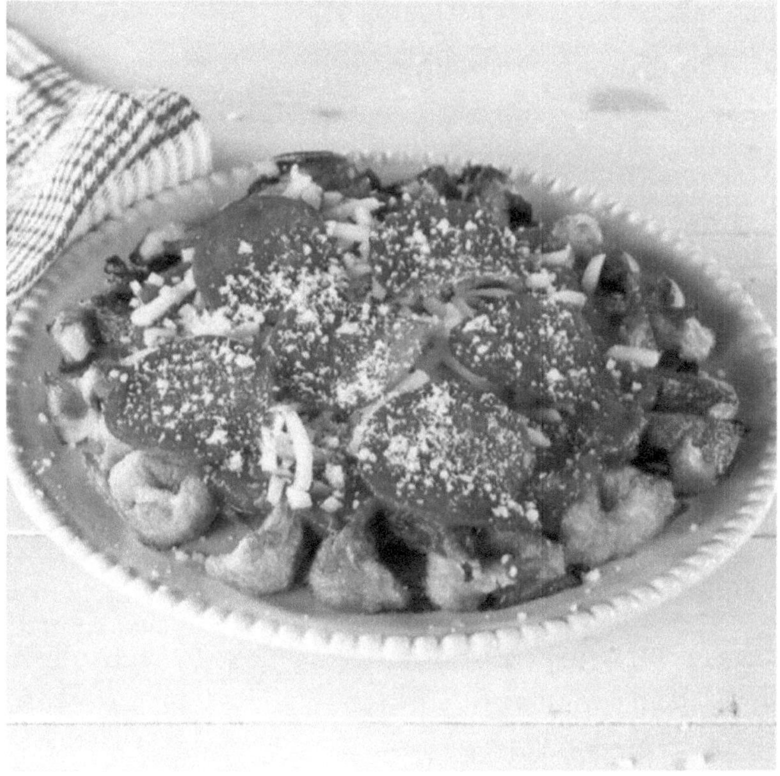

INGREDIENTS

FOR PIZZA CHAFFLES:

2 large eggs

2 tbsp. almond flour

1/2 tsp. kosher salt

1/2 tsp. baking soda

1 1/2 c. shredded mozzarella, divided

1/3 c. pepperoni slices

Freshly grated Parmesan, for serving

DIRECTIONS

Preheat waffle maker according to manufacturer's directions. In a medium bowl, whisk eggs, almond flour, salt, and baking soda together. Add 1 cup mozzarella and stir to coat.

Pour 1/2 cup mixture into center of waffle maker and cook until golden and crispy, 2 to 3 minutes. Repeat with remaining batter.

Immediately top with marinara, remaining ½ cup mozzarella, pepperoni, and a sprinkle of Parmesan.

Keto Garlic Bread

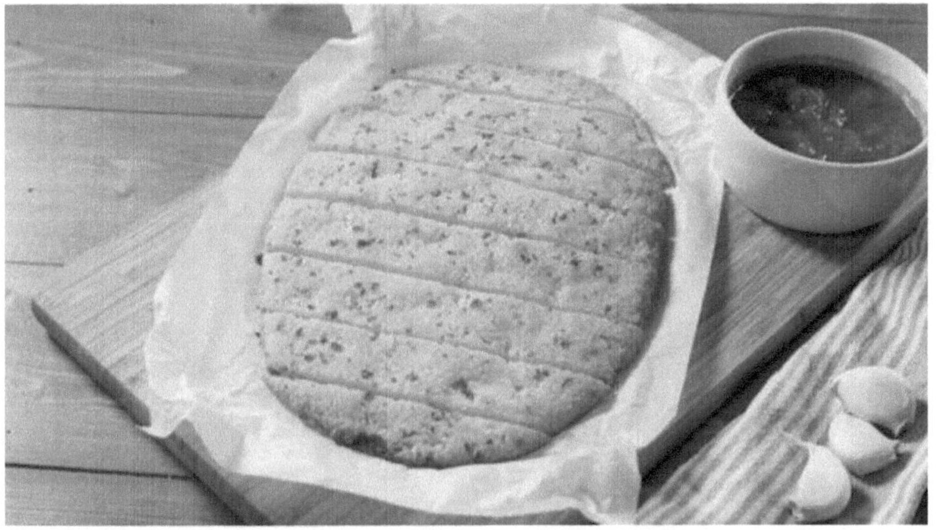

The secret to really good low-carb bread? Cheese, glorious cheese! Fun fact: The same concept applies to cauliflower crust.

INGREDIENTS

1 c. shredded mozzarella

1/2 c. finely ground almond flour

2 tbsp. cream cheese

1 tbsp. garlic powder

1 tsp. baking powder

Kosher salt

1 large egg

1 tbsp. butter, melted

1 clove garlic, minced

1 tbsp. freshly chopped parsley

1 tbsp. freshly grated Parmesan

Marinara, warmed, for serving

DIRECTIONS

Preheat oven to 400° and line a large baking sheet with parchment paper. In a medium, microwave-safe bowl, add mozzarella, almond flour, cream cheese, garlic powder, baking powder, and a large pinch of salt. Microwave on high until cheeses are melted, about 1 minute. Stir in egg.

Shape dough into a ½"-thick oval on baking sheet.

In a small bowl, mix melted butter with garlic, parsley, and Parmesan. Brush mixture over top of bread.

Bake until golden, 15 to 17 minutes. Slice and serve with marinara sauce for dipping.